I0428791

DIY Organic Lotion Recipes
Quick and Easy Homemade Lotions on the Go

Disclaimer and Terms of Use:

Effort has been made to ensure that the information in this book is accurate and complete, however, the author and the publisher do not warrant the accuracy of the information, text and graphics contained within the book due to the rapidly changing nature of science, research, known and unknown facts and internet. The Author and the publisher do not hold any responsibility for errors, omissions or contrary interpretation of the subject matter herein. This book is presented solely for motivational and informational purposes only.

Table of Contents

Introduction

Organic lotions are great alternatives compared to over the counter manufactured lotions from the store. They provide a cost saving solution for every day skin care. The only thing you basically need to know is what ingredients you need to use.

The overall process of making homemade lotion is pretty much the same no matter what recipe you're using. You basically need a base, essential oils for the scent, and other additives to make the lotion more nourishing.

The most common ingredients include Shea butter, beeswax, myrrh, almond oil, and coconut oil. They provide powerful moisturizing effects. Some of them also contain vitamins that are needed by the skin.

Hand butter basically acts as a layer of protection for the skin. Beeswax also makes the skin feel firmer. A bit of a warning though is that you should take care when handling essential oils.

They are aromatic and you should cover your face when you handle them. Don't put in too much or else the scent will overtake the scent of the other ingredients.

This book will basically show you how to make your own lotions at home without the use of harmful chemicals. Try them and save some money. You can make them right in the comfort of your own home.

Rose Flower Water Facial Lotion

This lotion is formulated for use in any skin type. Beyond that, it can also be used to keep your face cool during hot summers or any hot day. Please see warning at the end of this recipe in case you plan to use this natural facial lotion during summer.

If you prefer not to have any greasy films on your skin then kukui nut oil should be in your list. Recommended essential oils for this recipe include grapefruit, lavender, as well as geranium essential oil. It's basically up to you which essential oil you're going to use.

Ingredients:

a) Rose flower water (2.5 teaspoons)
b) Natural beeswax pellets unbleached; acts as an emulsifier (0.5 teaspoons)
c) Your choice of essential oils (e.g. 10 drops Lavender, 10 drops geranium, 2 drops grapefruit)
d) Organic kukui nut oil (7 teaspoons)

Optional Ingredient:

a) organic grape seed extract, preservative (1 drop)

How to Make It:

Combine the beeswax and all the oils you have selected. Place them in a double boiler. Set the mixture on low heat. Pour rose water in a different boiler. Heat the liquid on low heat.

Whip oils after they have melted. Add rose water one drop at a time while whipping. Continue mixing until you get a creamy consistency.

Warning: Don't use this natural facial lotion if you will be exposed to the sun. Note that some oils like grape seed oil are phototoxic.

This lotion has a lot of nourishing ingredients. It provides a lot of nutrients for the skin. It's also a great natural solution for your baby's diaper rash. If you're looking for a natural treatment for eczema, then this is a good natural alternative. It's also a good treatment for stretch marks.

Ingredients:

a) Almond oil (half a cup)
b) Coconut oil (about 1/4 cup)
c) Beeswax (1/4 cup)

Optional Ingredients:

a) Vitamin E oil (1 teaspoon)
b) Cocoa butter (2 tablespoons)
c) Any essential oil of your choice

How to Make It:

This natural homemade lotion is very easy to make. All you have to do is mix all the ingredients in a pot. Place the pot on a stove and turn the heat on low. Allow all the ingredients to melt and mix occasionally.

Once all the ingredients have blended well turn the heat off. Allow the mixture to cool for a few minutes. Pour the ingredients in a glass jar or any container of your choice.

Take note that this homemade lotion has a longer shelf life than many of the lotions in this book. It actually has a 6 month shelf life if you keep it in the fridge.

Homemade Lotion Bars

These lotion bars are easy to make and easy to store. Turning your all-natural lotion into bar form extends its shelf life. Best of all, they still have the same nourishing effect on your skin.

Ingredients:

a) Shea butter (1/3 cup)
b) Beeswax (1 cup)
c) Mango butter (1/3 cup)
d) Cocoa butter (1/3 cup)
e) Coconut oil (1 cup)

Optional Ingredients:

a) Vitamin E oil, preservative (1 teaspoon)

How to Make It:

Take note that this recipe can be adjusted according to your liking. You can even use any essential oil to add to the scent of each lotion bar. It's all just a matter of personal preference.

Combine all of the ingredients in the list. Place them in a container. If you're adding an essential oil, add that later. Grab a saucepan and pour in water up to an inch in depth. Boil water in saucepan. Place container in water to allow the ingredients to melt.

Stir the mixture constantly until it attains a smooth consistency. Remove container from boiling water and turn the heat off. Now you can add the essential oils of your choice.

Remember to stir everything gently. Pour the mixture into molds. Allow them to cool and harden. Pop the bars out of the mold only when they have hardened completely.

You can keep them in the molds overnight so you can be sure that they are already hard enough to pop out. Pop out the bars only when they're ready or else they come out in mashed up pieces.

Homemade Jojoba Moisturizing Lotion

The following is a base recipe for a homemade skin moisturizing lotion. The recipe may have recommended essential oils but you are free to make adjustments. You may use any essential oils that you prefer.

Ingredients:

    a) Shea butter (4 oz.)
    b) Jojoba oil (2 tablespoons)
    c) Lavender essential oil (15 drops)
    d) Rosemary essential oil (10 drops)
    e) Carrot seed oil (7 drops)
    f) Tea tree essential oil (3 drops)

How to Make It:

Heat a saucepan using low to medium heat. Don't get the pan too hot or else the ingredients will burn. Once the sauce pan gets hot enough, place Shea butter inside it and melt.

Once the entire batch of Shea butter is melted, add jojoba oil. Turn off the heat. Mix ingredients thoroughly.

When it has already been blended well, place the mixture into a bowl. Place the bowl inside your freezer for cooling. Keep it inside for 15 minutes or until the mixture becomes slightly solidified. Don't let it get as hard as a bar of soap. You shouldn't freeze the mixture too.

After 15 minutes, or once the mixture becomes solid looking, take it out of the freezer. Add in your essential oils. Using a wire whisk (or a food processor with a whisk attachment), give it a gentle whipping. Whip the mixture only for a couple of minutes.

Keep whipping until the mixture attains a creamy consistency. This usually takes only one to two minutes to make. After that, scoop the newly formulated moisturizing lotion into a jar or container. Store it at room temperature.

Simple Coconut Oil Lotion Recipe with Essential Oils

This is a very simple recipe and it only uses two ingredients. Remember that essential oils are very aromatic so you should wear a mask when you handle them.

Materials and Ingredients:

a) Coconut oil (4 jars – 16 oz. each)
b) Organic geranium oil (two bottles – 10 ml. each)
c) Organic lavender oil (two bottles – 10 ml. each)
d) glass jars (containers)

How to Make It:

Heat coconut oil in a pot over low heat until everything is dissolved into a liquid state. You can also do this by placing the coconut oil in a microwavable container and heating in the microwave for 90 seconds. If you use the microwave, make sure to remove the lids.

Add 1 teaspoon of an essential oil of your choice for each jar of coconut oil you have used. Use one jar for one type of oil. Stir the contents of each jar. Carefully pour the mixture into glass jars. Fill all the way up to a quarter inch from the top.

Cover each jar with its lid. Allow the jars to cool down to room temperature. Store them in a cool, dry place.

Tips:

Make sure to wash all the jars you're going to use. Make sure they are dry before you pour the mixtures. You can use only one essential oil scent or you can use both geranium and lavender. If you are using more than one scent of essential oil, make sure to label each jar so you know which scent is used for each jar.

Organic Eczema Treatment Body Butter Lotion

This next organic lotion recipe can be used as a type of treatment for eczema. However, even if you don't use it to treat that skin condition, it still provides a full-bodied feel and a nice nutty smell to it. It's a great relaxing lotion to cap off a long tiring day.

Coconut oil easily reminds people of the beach, which basically adds to the overall relaxing effect. Both the Shea butter as well as the almond oil content gives off that nutty smell.

Ingredients:

a) Organic Coconut Oil (4 ounces)
b) Organic Sweet Almond Oil (4 ounces)
c) Raw Shea Butter (8 ounces)
d) Frankincense essential oils (10 drops)

How to Make It:

This organic lotion recipe is very easy to make. All you have to do is to put everything in the list of ingredients above in a double boiler. Use low to medium heat. Both the Shea butter and coconut oil should be melted and stirred lightly.

Once both oils have blended, then turn the heat off. Allow the mixture to cool before transferring it into a container (preferably one made out of glass). Chill the mixture inside the fridge for about an hour.

After the mixture gets chilled, take it out of the fridge and whip it in an electric mixer. The idea is to create emulsion. Once the mixture has been emulsified, transfer the contents into a container with a lid.

Nourishing Hand and Body Cream

Coconut oil, cocoa butter, and Shea butter provide a moisturizing effect on the skin. They make a great hand and body lotion if you use them to make a natural lotion. Of course you should know just how much of every ingredient you should use.

Be careful when you buy Shea butter. If you use raw Shea butter, then you may end up with a hand a body lotion that will have a more liquid consistency. You can still use that kind of lotion but you will need a container that has a pump on the lid.

Orange essence signals relaxation to the brain. You can use this hand and body lotion after a quick shower. It can also be used before going to bed at night.

Ingredients:

a) Coconut oil (1/4 cup)
b) Shea butter (1/8 cup)
c) Cocoa butter (1/8 cup)
d) Aloe Vera juice (1 tablespoon)
e) Sweet almond oil or you can use jojoba oil as a substitute (1 tablespoon)
f) Orange essential oil (5 drops)

How to Make It:

Place the coconut oil, Shea butter, and cocoa butter in a pan. Heat all these ingredients using low heat. Make sure that everything is melted. Remove the pan from the heat.

Mix essential oils, liquid oils from the pan, and essential oils. Stir them well to combine all ingredients. Allow the ingredients to cool down to room temperature. Transfer contents into small canning jars.

Basic Homemade Organic Lotion

This homemade organic lotion leaves your skin really soft. Some people may think that it feels a little too oily. If that is the case that only means you didn't give the mixture enough whipping using a mixer.

Note that the step that requires you to chill the oil mixture is essential to create that creamy texture. Make sure that the blended oils get chilled and slightly solidified before you attempt to whip it.

You can purchase the gentle baby essential oil blend from the store or make it yourself. It's made from a combination of several essential oils, namely: coriander, geranium, lemon, jasmine, palmarosa, ylang, roman chamomile, rose, and rosewood. The gentle baby essential oil blend gives this lotion a nice refreshing scent.

Note that some ingredients have been labeled as optional. You can still make this lotion recipe without them. However, if you really want to get that unique scent and texture on your skin then those ingredients become highly recommended.

Ingredients:

    a) Beeswax (1 1/2 tablespoons)
    b) Cocoa butter (1 cup)
    c) Almond oil (1/2 cup)
    d) Coconut oil (1/2 cup

Optional Ingredients:

    a) Gentle Baby blend essential oil (5 drops)
    b) Pure Aloe Vera gel (skin protection) (1 tablespoon)
    c) Non-nano zinc oxide (thickening agent) (1 tablespoon)

How to Make It:

Melt beeswax, Shea butter, almond oil, and coconut oil over medium heat. After all of these ingredients have melted and blended, store the mixture in the fridge for about an hour and half and allow it to cool.

Place the cooled oil blend into a mixer. Add non-nano zinc oxide, gentle baby blend, and Aloe Vera gel. Whip the entire mixture for five to ten minutes or until the concoction attains a nice whipped cream texture.

Organic Anti-Aging Facial Lotion

This anti-aging facial lotion makes use of honey and beeswax. These two ingredients are part and parcel of many beauty treatments. Some even laud their anti-aging properties.

Both of these primary ingredients act as natural moisturizers for the skin. They are in fact natural humectants, which helps the skin to retain moisture. It can even help to replenish the skin's moisture content.

Shea butter on the other hand gives the skin its elastic properties. Rosewater on the other hand helps to rejuvenate the skin. It also provides a good amount of skin toning. Remember to use jars with lids on top for proper storage.

Ingredients

    a) Organic Shea butter (2 tablespoons)
    b) Essential oils (choose your favorite!) (8 drops only)
    c) Wheat germ oil (4 teaspoons)
    d) Pure, organic beeswax (4 teaspoons)
    e) Organic honey (2 teaspoons)
    f) Rosewater (2 tablespoons)

How to Make It:

Grab a baking pan. Fill it with two inches of water. Place the pan with water on low to medium heat.

Grab a mixing bowl. Place the beeswax in mixing bowl. Place the bowl in a baking pan that has warm water in it. Allow beeswax to melt slowly. Stir it occasionally. This will help make the beeswax pearls to melt completely.

While waiting for the beeswax to melt, place rosewater in a cup. Place the cup in the warm water as well beside the bowl. Add Shea butter to the beeswax. Stir continuously until both the beeswax and Shea butter melt and blend together.

Add sweet almond oil and stir. Stir in wheat germ oil. Using a stick blender, give the mixture some light whipping. Make sure that all the ingredients have blended well.

Add rosewater and honey. Remove the blended mixture from heat. Stir the mixture continuously until it has cooled down to room temperature.

Add essential oils. For best anti-aging effects, jasmine, lavender, or sandalwood essential oils are recommended. Store the facial lotion in a glass container.

Vegan Facial Lotion

Ingredients:

a) Organic sweet almond oil (1/4 cup)
b) Organic olive oil (1/4 cup)
c) Neroli essential oil (8 drops)
d) Carnauba wax (1/16 cup)
e) Organic coconut oil (1/16 cup)
f) Organic grape seed oil (1/4 cup)
g) Vitamin e oil (1/4 teaspoon)
h) Organic aloe vera gel (1/2 cup)
i) Organic rose hydrosol (1 cup)

How to Make It:

Place all the oils in a glass saucepan. Warm them over very low heat. Allow the oils to get warmed thoroughly until they get melted. Stir the ingredients to prevent the oils from burning.

Once the oils have melted, remove them from heat and allow them to cool to room temperature.

Heat carnauba wax in a different saucepan. Use low heat as well. Make sure that the carnauba wax melts thoroughly. Set aside to cool.

Mix Aloe Vera gel and hydrosol in a separate container. Swish these ingredients gently.

Preheat a double broiler over very low flame. Pour half of the oil mixture inside. Add a quarter ounce of the melted wax. Stir them slowly until blended.

Place vitamin E oil and 6 ounces of the aloe-hydrosol blended mixture in a food processor. Add essential oil. Give it a good whipping until the ingredients have blended well.

Add the wax and oil mixture slowly. Keep blending until all the ingredients emulsify. Repeat the last few steps to make use of the remaining ingredients. Spoon the lotion into container. This natural lotion mixture can last for one year if stored well in the fridge.

Simple Whipped Body Butter Lotion

This recipe is for a simple body butter or lotion. Take note that it will remain in its white whipped state in cooler places. If you live in a place with warmer climate then you will have to store this homemade lotion in the fridge.

Ingredients:

   a) cocoa butter (1 cup)
   b) mild olive oil (1/2 cup)
   c) coconut oil (1/2 cup)

How to Make It:

Melt coconut oil and cocoa butter in a container. Remember to use low to medium heat. Stir the two oils together slowly and allow the smallest bits to melt into liquid form.

Stir in mild olive oil into the mixture. Chill the mixture in the fridge for several hours until it becomes semi-solid or slightly firm.

When the mixture solidifies slightly, put it in a standing mixer. Whip it up until it begins to form white peaks. Once the emulsified mixture has been whipped, scoop the up and transfer to a container with lid. Chill the whipped body butter in the fridge for another hour before using.

Winter Time Hand Lotion

Do you always get dry skin during the colder times of the year? Do you hate spending money on hand lotions or cream that only work for a little bit? This little recipe might help you with that.

Human skin naturally gets dry during winter or fall. Whenever it's cold outside, expect that your skin will feel slightly dryer. It's okay for some people but it can sometimes be a painful and itchy experience for others.

This simple recipe takes advantage of the health benefits of avocado, coconut, and beeswax. This is an all-natural concoction that keeps you free of synthetic chemicals that act as endocrine disruptors. It's a good remedy for dry or even cracked skin on the hands and arms; and it's budget friendly too!

Ingredients:

a) organic coconut oil (1/3 cup)
b) grated beeswax (1/8 cup)
c) organic avocado oil (1/4 cup)
d) essential oil of your choice
e) Aloe Vera cream or extract

How to Make It:

Place coconut oil, beeswax, and avocado oil a container. Place over medium heat. Stir occasionally to ensure that all the ingredients in the container are melted completely. Make sure there are no solid particles remaining.

Add the essential oil of your choice. Blend in Aloe Vera. Heat the mixture until everything inside the container and heat until everything is completely dissolved.

Set the mixture aside. Let it cool. Once it reaches room temperature you can store it in the fridge for three hours. After that, whip the mixture in a blender for five minutes or until it looks like whipped cream.

Store in jars for three hours and it will solidify even in room temperature. This natural lotion needs to be stored in the fridge or else it will spoil.

Gardener's Hand Lotion

This organic lotion recipe is specially formulated to care for tired working hands. If you love to work in your garden all day or if you work with your hands to earn your hard earned cash then this hand lotion will be a good reward at the end of the day. It's very easy to make and it soothes the skin on your hands.

Ingredients:

a) Cedarwood essential oil (10 drops)
b) Shea butter (1/4 cup)
c) Beeswax (1 tablespoon)
d) Myrrh essential oil (10 drops)
e) Sweet almond oil (1/8 cup)

Instructions:

Place the sweet almond oil, Shea butter, and beeswax in a Pyrex cup or similar container. Melt them in low heat. Stir occasionally until all the ingredients blend well. Remove from heat. Set aside and let it cool for 15 minutes.

Add myrrh essential oil and sweet almond oil. Stir well to get them blended in. Pour the mixture a glass container. Store for several hours until the mixture hardens completely.

Apply the hand butter to your dry hands as often as needed–especially after a long day working outside or playing in the dirt. This recipe makes a woodsy scent, which gardeners and nature lovers will easily recognize.

Herb Enhanced Hand Lotion

This is another natural hand lotion that you can use to soothe tired hands. It is vitamin and herb enriched. If you don't like the smell of coconut oil, you can replace it with cocoa butter instead.

Ingredients:

a) Almond oil (1/2 cup)
b) Coconut oil (1/4 cup)
c) Beeswax (1/4 cup)

Additional Ingredients:

a) Vitamin E oil (1 teaspoon)
b) Shea butter (2 tablespoons)
c) Your preferred essential oils
d) Vanilla extract or other natural extracts
e) A pinch of your preferred herbs (powder form)

How to Make It:

Combine all the ingredients in the list above in jar or container that's big enough. Get a saucepan and fill it with an inch of water. Heat the saucepan using medium heat. Place the jar in saucepan.

Stir the ingredients in the jar occasionally. Make sure that all the ingredients are blended evenly. Once the ingredients are well incorporated, set the jar aside to cool.

Transfer the contents of the jar in the container you intend to store it in. This herb enhanced hand lotion will store for more than six months if you keep it in the fridge.

Honey Enriched Facial Cold Cream

Honey is a staple for many anti-aging solutions. It makes a good facial mask to peel away your face's old skin. This particular facial lotion is safe for use in the face. It leaves your skin refreshed after use.

Ingredients:

a) Cold-pressed safflower oil (3 tablespoons)
b) Honey (1 teaspoon)
c) Grated beeswax (2 teaspoons)
d) Distilled water (3 tablespoons)

How to Make It:

Grab a small container. Place over low heat. Place the beeswax and safflower oil inside and stir occasionally. Stir until the safflower and beeswax melt and blend together.

When the mixture has melted, remove it from the heat. Drizzle the honey slowly one small amount at a time. Beat the mixture as you add the honey.

After that, add water one small amount at a time while continuously beating the mixture. Let the mixture sit. Notice that the cold cream and the water will separate.

The honey-enriched cold cream will tend to float. Once that occurs, drain the water. Store the facial cream in a glass container. Keep it refrigerated to extend its shelf life.

Ready to Make Vitamin E Creamy Lotion

This is a basic vitamin E based organic lotion recipe. It provides natural nourishment that you can apply to your skin where you need it the most. You can use your regular vitamin E capsules as the main additive to this creamy lotion.

This is an easy to make concoction and you can make a small batch in less than five minutes. It can be included in any nightly ritual. You can also use it right after you wash makeup off your face.

Ingredients:

a) 3 Vitamin E capsules (equivalent of 300 units)
b) Honey (1/2 teaspoon)
c) Plain yoghurt (2 teaspoons)
d) Lemon juice (1/2 teaspoon)

How to Make It:

Mix the lemon juice, yogurt, and honey in a small bowl. Open three vitamin E capsules and place the contents in the middle of the mixture. Fold the vitamin E until it is thoroughly blended in the cream.

Massage this facial lotion gently on your face. Leave it on for about 15 minutes. Store the remaining cream in the fridge. It will have a maximum shelf life of 4 days when it is refrigerated.

Ready to Make Anti-Wrinkle Cream

This ready to make facial lotion and anti-wrinkle cream smells good enough to eat. Well, it's not actually formulated for your belly but it will do wonders for tired stressed skin. If you've been out on the road all day exposed to the sun and air pollution, this facial cream and lotion will be a huge relief for your skin.

Ingredients:

a) Apple juice (1 teaspoon)
b) Lemon juice (1 teaspoon)
c) Lime juice (1 teaspoon)
d) Buttermilk (2 tablespoons)
e) Rosemary leaves (1 tablespoon)
f) Grapes (3 seedless)
g) Pear (1/4)
h) Egg Whites (from 2 eggs)

How to Make It:

This ready to make lotion can be made in just about five minutes, which includes the preparation time. All need to do is to get your blender out. Place all the ingredients inside.

Set your blender to medium speed. The next step is to blender all the ingredients for only half a minute. Scoop up the emulsified mixture and place it in a dry clean container.

Right then and there facial lotion is ready to use. Dab a small amount of this cream on your face especially on the wrinkles. Allow it to dry and then rinse your face using warm water.

You can then follow it up with a natural homemade moisturizer. This anti-wrinkle lotion will have a shelf life of up to four days when stored in the fridge.

Dry Skin Cream on the Go

Pressed for time and always in a hurry? This ready to make lotion and cream is a quick treatment for dry skin. You can make this concoction in less than 10 minutes.

Remember that it's only a quick solution for dry skin in case you're in a hurry. It will help a bit but you will need a much longer treatment at the end of the day.

Ingredients:

a) Grated beeswax (2 tablespoons)
b) Vitamin E oil (2 teaspoons)
c) Sesame seed oil (1/2 cup)
d) Grapefruit essential oil (3 drops)
e) Water (1/2 cup)

How to Make It:

Mix sesame oil, beeswax, and vitamin E oil in a Pyrex cup or any similar container. Place it over a stove with low heat. Melt the oils and stir as needed. When they have been melted blended well, remove the mixture from the heat.

In a separate container, heat the grapefruit essential oil and water over low heat. Once some steam comes up from the water and essential oil mixture, remove it from the heat.

Combine both mixtures in a separate container. Mix them well until everything blends evenly. Let it cool for a few minutes. When it is cool enough, you can use it directly on your skin.

Ginger Facial Lotion

If you love the smell of ginger then this facial lotion and cream will be perfect for you. It gives off an Asian scent, which is nice and refreshing. It's a great alternative for over the counter creams.

Ingredients:

a) Apricot kernel oil (2 teaspoons)
b) Cocoa butter (1/2 cup)
c) Light sesame oil (2 teaspoons)
d) Fresh ginger (5cm piece)
e) Vitamin E oil (2 teaspoons)

How to Make It:

Grate the ginger into fine pieces. Squeeze the pieces to get ginger juice, which will be about $1/8^{th}$ of a teaspoon full. Another alternative is to use a mortar and pestle.

Yet another option is to use a masticating juicer but you will need a lot more ginger than the amount specified in this recipe. Alternatively, if you can buy all natural ginger extract from the store then you can use that instead.

Place the ginger juice as well as the rest of the ingredients into a jar. Heat the ingredients using low heat until the cocoa butter melts completely. Pour mixture into a dry container. Store the lotion in a cool dry place. You can apply this lotion on your face and all over your neck.

Aloe Vera Face Cream

Aloe Vera is known for its healthy skin benefits. Fresh Aloe Vera extract is a refreshing moisturizer for tired old skin. Using it as a facial lotion will achieve this effect. It also provides a lot of needed nourishment.

Ingredients:

a) Coconut oil (1/3 cup)
b) Distilled water (2/3 cup)
c) Grated beeswax (2 tablespoons)
d) Aloe Vera gel (1/3 cup)
e) Apricot oil (3/4 cup)
f) Essential oil of your choice (2 drops)
g) Lanolin (1/4 teaspoon)
h) Vitamins A and E extract

How to Make It:

Combine the vitamins A and E, Aloe Vera gel, water, and essential oils in a cup. Mix beeswax, the different oils, and lanolin in a small pot and heat them up in a low heat. Remove the mixture off the heat when they have all melted completely.

Allow the mixture to cool down to room temperature. Place all the ingredients in a blender. Blend them using a high-speed setting. Make sure to pour the water mixture little by little as you blend.

Keep blending until you achieve a creamy texture. It will come out quite thick. Keep this mixture in the fridge since it doesn't have any preservatives.

Green Tea Face Lotion and Cleanser

Green tea is a great facial cleanser. It will deep-cleans the skin. After rinsing this lotion off your face remember to apply a moisturizer.

Ingredients:

a) Aloe Vera juice (2 tablespoons)
b) Citric acid (1 teaspoon)
c) Emulsifying wax (2 tablespoons)
d) Green tea (1/2 cup)
e) Vitamin e (4 capsules)
f) Hazelnut oil (4 tablespoons)

Ingredients:

If you do not have Aloe Vera juice you can blend a couple of stalks of Aloe Vera and then just strain the juice. Grab a glass bowl and mix the emulsifying wax and the hazelnut oil.

Fill a saucepan with an inch of water. Heat the water in low heat and place the glass bowl and heat the mixture inside. While that is heating up brew your green tea in half a cup of water.

Add the green tea extract to the glass bowl. After that set the mixture aside and allow it too cool. Add vitamin E only after the mixture cools. Add citric acid. Mix it well and then place in your storage container.

Unscented Homemade Facial Lotion

This homemade facial lotion is called "unscented." Well, you should take that with a grain of salt. It's unscented simply because this recipe does not include any essential oils.

It will have a blend of coconut and cocoa butter smell, but it won't be too strong. Come to think of it, the scent of this facial cream is actually quite refreshing.

Ingredients:

a) Extra-virgin olive oil (½ tablespoon)
b) Cocoa butter (2½ tablespoons)
c) Coconut oil (1 tablespoon)

How to Make It:

Heat an inch of water in a pan. Make sure the water is about an inch in depth. Use low medium heat. Place the coconut oil in a container that will fit inside the pan. Place the container in the pan to melt the coconut oil.

Place the rest of the ingredients inside the container with the coconut oil. Make sure that all the ingredients have melted completely. Keep stirring every now and then to make sure all the ingredients blend completely.

Remove the mixture from the heat. Set it aside to cool a bit. Once it has cooled, place the mixture in a container that has a lid. Shake the contents and then let it sit.

Note that if you make this lotion during winter, it will actually solidify if you leave it out. It's usually creamy the rest of the year.

Vitamin E Enhanced All Natural Lotion

This recipe is for a powerfully enhanced vitamin E lotion. It's really easy to make but it will take some time to prepare all the ingredients. After getting all the necessary things ready, making the mixture is really quick.

Ingredients:

a) Almond oil (1/4 cup)
b) Vitamin E oil (3/4 tablespoon)
c) Cocoa butter (1/2 cup)
d) Grated beeswax (2 teaspoon)
e) Unrefined coconut oil (1/2 cup)

How to Make It:

Place all the ingredients in a container that's large enough. Place an inch of water in a pan and allow the water to boil. Place the container in the boiling water to heat the ingredients inside.

Melt all the ingredients thoroughly. Stir every once in a while. Once the ingredients have melted give it one last stir and then set the mixture aside. Place the mixture in a lidded container and allow it to cool. You can use this vitamin-enhanced lotion as soon as it has cooled completely.

Deep Cleansing Organic Facial Lotion

This is one of the few deep cleansing solutions in this book. Here's an important tip: after using this lotion, rinse it off and use moisturizer on your face. Some people might feel that it leaves their face a bit dry.

Ingredients:

a) Vitamin E oil (half a teaspoon)
b) Almond oil (6 tablespoons)
c) Sandalwood water (2/3 cup)
d) Shea butter (3 tablespoons)
e) Coconut oil (2 tablespoons)
f) Vanilla extract (1 teaspoon)
g) Beeswax (1 tablespoon)
h) Aloe Vera gel (1/3 cup)
i) Cacao butter (¼ cup)
j) Patchouli essential oil (10 drops)

How to Make It:

Melt coconut oil, Shea butter, beeswax, and cacao butter in a double boiler. While that is melting, mix sandalwood water and the Aloe Vera gel in another container. When oils are melted set them aside to cool.

Add the oils to a blender plus the almond oil. Blend thoroughly using low seed. After that you should stream in the sandalwood water plus Aloe Vera while blending.

Blend the mixture for 3 minutes or until the cream becomes thick. Add the vanilla, vitamin E, and essential oils. Keep blending until everything is incorporated into the lotion completely. Place the all-natural lotion in a lidded container. Remember to store it in the fridge for a longer shelf life.

Homemade Lotion for Kings

This homemade lotion is made from myrrh and frankincense. These ingredients mainly hydrate the skin. It also nourishes the skin with essential vitamins and other essential nutrients.

Ingredients:

a) Frankincense essential oil (15 drops)
b) Olive oil (1/4 cup)
c) Coconut oil (1/4 cup)
d) Bees wax (1/4 cup)
e) Shea butter (1/4 cup)
f) Vitamin E (2 tablespoon)
g) Myrrh essential oil (15 drops)

How to Make It:

Combine beeswax, Shea butter, olive oil, and coconut oil, in a bowl. Place the bowl in a pan or container with water. Alternatively you can use a double broiler. Use medium heat to melt the oil and other ingredients.

When the ingredients have melted, place the mixture in the fridge for several hours so that it will solidify. Place solidified mixture in a blender and blend it at medium speed. Beat the mixture until it is thick and fluffy.

Add vitamin E plus essential oils and mix well. Place the mixture in a lidded container. You can store this lotion in a cool dry place.

Conclusion

Making and using organic lotion recipes can be incorporated into anyone's daily routine. The ingredients are easy to find and some of them are can be found in most grocery stores. You just have to take the time to include them in your next shopping trip.

After you have tried all the recipes included here you can experiment and make your own recipes. You can mix and match different waxes and oils. You can also experiment with different essential oils when you try to make your own recipes.

Remember that the different formulations of every recipe mentioned here serve different purposes. Using them regularly will eventually save you money while getting your skin nourished.